Finding the Cure

NATTO

VICTORIA BELL, RN

NATTO
Finding the Cure
VICTORIA BELL, RN

Printed in the United States of America

ISBN-13: **978-** 1096503682

MEDICAL DISCLAIMER

Victoria Bell, RN does not diagnose, treat or prevent any medical conditions; instead she helps people get healthy mentally, physically and spiritually. Information provided is not designed to take the place of or provide medical advice, professional diagnosis, opinion, treatment or services to you or to any other individual. Victoria Bell, RN, is not liable or responsible for any advice, course of treatment, diagnosis or any other information, services or product you obtain through any information created or distributed by her.

RELIGIOUS DISCLAIMER

Please note that this book is filled with scriptures Holy Spirit used to teach and comfort me. Please seek Holy Spirit's guidance on what He wants to teach and emphasized for you.

NAME CHANGES

YAHUAH is used for God or Our Heavenly Father's name and Yahowashi for the only begotten son or "Christ Jesus" in King James Version Bibles. I do not claim to know all and am not advocating for anyone else to call them by these names. We are all to be led by the Holy Spirit whatsoever He tells us, so do.

INTRODUCTION

I am so utterly dependent upon my Lord Yahowashi HaMashiach to teach me all things. I pray that He will guide and use me to live and teach the truth of His Holiness so that we can all be free in His Name.

[AND]. . . the Holy Ghost . . . SHALL TEACH YOU ALL THINGS, and bring ALL THINGS to your REMEMBRANCE, *whatsoever I have said unto you.*

John 14:26

20 For the INVISIBLE THINGS *of* **Him** *from the creation of the world* **are clearly seen, BEING UNDERSTOOD BY THE THINGS THAT ARE MADE,** *even* **His ETERNAL POWER** *and Godhead;* **SO THAT THEY ARE WITHOUT EXCUSE!**

Romans 1:20

And ye shall **KNOW the TRUTH,** *AND* **the TRUTH** *shall* **MAKE you FREE!**

John 8:32

We Believe in Miracles
Because We Believe in YAHUAH!
HalleluYAH!!

Chapter 1

WHAT IS THE CURE FOR CANCER?

How many cures for cancer are there?

How many people have cancer?

That is how many cures there are and that goes for every sickness and DIS-EASE including injuries, etc.

All I can tell you is what works for me at this moment in time. Otherwise, I am completely dependent upon the Holy One to lead and guide me to my healing. HalleluYAH? HalleluYAH!

It's Obedience, brothers and sisters, that guides us to that one cure especially designed for us by the Holy One. HalleluYAH!

It's OBEDIENCE, brothers and sisters, that guides us to that one cure especially designed for us by the Holy One. HalleluYAH!

It's Righteous Living, giving up the Pleasures of the Flesh and the Ways of the World.

It's giving up eating animal sacrifices. No living creature that YAHUAH breathed life into is fit for consumption. Please read the Gospel of the Holy Twelve.

Didn't YAHUAH let the Israelites after they left Egypt eat flesh and even provided abundant quail for them to eat because they complained of the manna? But afterward made them to suffer and die because of their LUST for FLESH?

> 31 And there went forth a wind from the LORD, and brought quails from the sea, and let them fall by the camp . . .
> 32 And the people . . . gathered the quails . . .
> 33 And while the flesh was yet between their teeth, ere it was chewed, **the wrath of the LORD was kindled against the people**, and **the LORD smote the people with a VERY GREAT PLAGUE**.
> 34 And he called the name of that place Kibrothhattaavah: **BECAUSE** there they buried **THE PEOPLE** that **LUSTED**.
> **Numbers 11:21-24**

And nobody seems to be talking about the curse YAHUAH gave to the decendants of Noah after the flood for eating meat. Yes, He said they could but that it comes with a price, and that price is DEATH!

> ³ Every moving thing that liveth shall be meat for you; even as the green herb have I given you all things.
> ⁴ BUT FLESH with the life thereof, which is the BLOOD thereof, **SHALL YE NOT EAT**.

[HOW MANY OF YOU LIKE YOUR MEAT UNDERCOOKED? NOW HERE'S THE CURSE. . .]

> ⁵ **AND SURELY YOUR BLOOD OF YOUR LIVES WILL I REQUIRE;** *AT THE HAND OF EVERY BEAST WILL I REQUIRE IT,* and at the hand of man; at the hand of every man's brother will I require the life of man.
> **Genesis 9:3-5**

Meaning, our blood is required for every beast that we kill. We give our life away each time we eat meat. Scientifically, there is evidence to show that our bodies are not made to eat meat; our intestinal tract is too long and narrow for adequate digestion, are teeth are too dull and flat for the tearing of it. In fact, it is proven that meat does not digest but rather ferments creating ammonia and an acidic environment unconducive to health.

We are supposed to hear, listen and obey the Holy One but if we are not living righteously and living on compulsory or addictive behaviors, meaning we have NO self-control, we are not going to be hearing from the holy One but the one who likes to lead us astray to the lusts of the flesh. HalleluYAH!

The lifestyle of the World just set us up to live in fear because you know deep down inside that you are doing wrong. That's why most people seek out man i.e. doctors first for their medicine instead of the Holy One because they don't want to admit to God that they are living their lives selfishly and unholy. Nobody does!

> If my people, which are called by my name, shall humble themselves, and pray, and seek my face, and turn from their wicked ways; then will I hear from heaven, and will forgive their sin, and will heal their land [meaning their bodies as well].
>
> **2 Chronicles 7:14**

I can't help but bring to you this message. I have been suppressing it ever since I gave my life over to the Lord about six years ago. I had to become more holy and give-up more of the ways of this world before I could. And it's by the strength of the Holy One living inside me that even makes this possible. I couldn't do it otherwise. No one can. It's an illusion if they think so.

He also give me the words to speak. I cannot do this on my own. I was raised a "cowherd" just like most everybody else. But I was born to overcome this people pleasing illness everyone seems to have succumbed to. We hate being prisoners of our own mind. We want to break free to please the Holy One who is above and within. We all do. We hate being suppressed and controlled by the wicked forces of this World.

Nevertheless,

Remember the word that I said unto you, the servant is not greater than his lord. If they have persecuted me, they will also persecute you; if they have kept my saying, they will keep yours also.
John 15:20

34 Think not that I am come to send peace on earth: I came not to send peace, but a sword.
35 For I am come to set a man at variance against his father, and the daughter against her mother, and the daughter in law against her mother in law.
36 **And a man's foes shall be they of his own household.**
37 HE THAT LOVETH father or mother MORE THAN ME **IS NOT WORTHY OF**

ME: and HE THAT LOVETH son or daughter MORE THAN ME **IS NOT WORTHY OF ME.**

38 And HE THAT TAKETH NOT his cross, and followeth after me, **IS NOT WORTHY OF ME**.

39 He that findeth his life **[meaning living to his own pleasure and will]** shall lose it: and he that loseth his life **[meaning stops living for self and by his own will and ideas]** for my sake shall find it.

40 He that receiveth you receiveth me, and he that receiveth me receiveth him that sent me. **HalleluYAH?!**

Matthew 10:37-40

If ye were of the world, the world would love his own **[He chose us, we didn't chose Him]** BUT BECAUSE ye are NOT of the WORLD, **BUT I HAVE CHOSEN YOU** out of the world, **THEREFORE THE WORLD HATETH YOU. [Guaranteed if you are living your life for YAHUAH!]**

John 15:19

Regardless of what you believe, I believe we all know that the Spiritual Realm is real. There are too many miraculous "coincidences" to be otherwise. And if this be so, then the food we eat matters because it carries with it the life and death it had to feed your belly. At least think of it this way to help make better choices for your health and recovery to health. HalleluYAH?!

Chapter 2

WHY JAPANESE NATTO?

How many of us believe we are at DIS-EASE due to some lack of medication or surgery?

> *"No man, person, or "education" system drummed up by the ruling powers of this world was ever created to help man realize that he are Powerful Spiritual Beings able to heal oneself when given the will to do so."*
>
> Anonymous

There are still remnants of ancient wisdom where societies have been virtually untouched by the modern health practices of western society. Okinawa, Japan is one such place where healthy centurions are common but life expectancy is gradually decreasing as their diet changes to include more rice and fat to match that of the modern Japanese diet. However, the risk of cardiac disease, cancers, and other DIS-EASE that plague modern civilizations such as here in the States are practically unheard of.

Their total flesh intake is very low and it does not come from poorly run factory farms. The average total amount of flesh is about 17 pounds per annum.

They also have the notion of eating more food with a lower caloric intake and only eating until you are 80 per cent full. About 30% of the calories come from green and yellow vegetables and their main staple is a purple-fleshed sweet potato.

Japanese are also known to eat more than 12 grams of salt per day, unlike the meager 2 grams recommended by the Allopathic Health Care System. Sea Salt provides the minerals essential for bone building.

Perhaps even more importantly, is the fact that they do not live or eat as the rest of the world does.

One of the most important soy products that the majority of the Japanese eat is a soy product called NATTO.

NATTO are cooked soybeans fermented with **Bacillus subtilis** or **Bacillus natto**. **Bacillus natto** is one of the bacterial champions that secretes an **alkaline** protease enzyme. Therefore, NATTO is a potent antifungal, antitumor, fibrin clot inhibitor, anti-parasitic, antimicrobial, and anti-inflammatory. Most importantly, the enzyme action helps accelerate chemical reactions for new bone formation.

Why is new bone formation so important?

Our bones create our immune system. They also create our red blood cells and stem cells to provide the building blocks for ALL bone and tissue preplacement and repair. It helps to protect our brain, heart, and other organs from injury from attacks from internal parasites, viruses and bacteria. Without healthy bones, we are sitting ducks for the next opportune DIS-EASE, sickness, or injury.

Now, I am NOT saying everyone should take NATTO. Those on blood thinning medications should definitely be more cautious consuming Natto as it is a natural blood thinner. I recommend that everyone consult your physician and seek the advice of Holy Spirit when determining whether this food would be a good solution for you.

That being said, NATTO is known to clear blood of impurities, dissolves blood clots, clear arteries, and other fibrin causing Alzheimer's.

NATTO has many micronutrients such as Calcium, Manganese, Zinc, Copper, and Selenium, which are all important components for bone health.

NATTO is the only vegetarian source of Vitamin K2 and has more than three times as much K2 than any other source and 100 times more than cheese. This Vitamin is required to assimilate Calcium and other minerals into the bone.

NATTO improves digestion. Our body contains trillions of microorganisms, more than the number of cells in your body. Natto acts as a probiotic to defend against harmful bacteria in your gut and body. Probiotics can help reduce constipation, gas, diarrhea, and help heal Inflammatory Bowel Disease and other colon related diseases.

NATTO helps alkalize the body. Blood pH plays a critical role in the prevention and treatment of cancer. Cancer is associated with an acidic body chemistry. The American diet with all the unhealthy foods, snacks, fast foods, processed foods, sodas **and overeating** create acid so that the body has to draw upon the bone minerals such as Calcium to keep your body from dying. Over the years of perpetual abuse and neglect, the bones become depleted and our immune system becomes crippled, and we become vulnerable acute and chronic illness and injuries.

However, NATTO may be an acquired taste. Some people are unable to get past the ammonia-like smell, flavor, or the slimy-sticky-stringy texture. I find this especially true if they use unpleasant words to describe it. Words have more power than most people realize.

When I first watched a video on NATTO, I did not know if I could eat it but when I saw how the Japanese spoke loving words to their NATTO, I thought I would give it a try. So I started saying things like "I love NATTO" just as the Japanese did and Holy Spirit gave me the ability to enjoy this food right from the start. HalleluYAH!

Probably, even more importantly, is it's not so much of what you eat that makes you healthier but what you don't eat. Foods such as:

- Bread, pastry, flour

- Coffee & Tea, anything with caffeine

- Carbonated drinks

- Sugar and sugar substitutes

- Meat and Dairy

Create an acid environment in the gut which feed acid-forming fungi. These fungi then create cravings for more of the same to self-propagate.

Most people are unwilling or unable to give up these addictive, habit forming foods. When foods acidify the body, the body is forced to rob your bones of nutrients thus making your body vulnerable to bacteria, fungi, viruses, sickness, dis-ease, and injury.

Unfortunately, instead of giving up these damaging habit forming foods and changing their ways to eating for their health, one usually goes to the "doctor" to receive a "pill" or have "surgery" to get rid of any symptoms they might have. They would rather do anything than to admit they have been living in the "Lust of the Flesh" or basically living a lie.

The word Pharmakeia is defined by:
Strong's Concordance

pharmakeia: (far-mak-i'-ah) φαρμακεία, ας, ἡ Noun, Feminine

the use of medicine, drugs or spells

Definition: **magic, sorcery, enchantment.**
HELPS Word-studies

5331 *pharmakeía* (from *pharmakeuō*, "administer drugs") – properly, **drug-related sorcery, like the practice of magical-arts, etc.** (A. T. Robertson).

However, the pill or surgery only covers the symptoms temporarily at best until the next symptom or symptoms occur. Changing the way we live is the only solution to a problem or problems will continue to manifest.

I hate to say it, but I believe every problem, great or small, even if it appears to be of a spiritual nature by our refusal to serve YAHUAH and not forsaking our own Lusts or Pride of Life. I could go into some scriptures here but I think everyone knows the validity of this to be true. If not, they just don't want to admit it. I am just telling you how I see it. We all want to be well but we don't want to give up the ways of this world. HalleluYAH!

So if you want to be righteous and holy and well, you have to give up the ways of this world. I can do nothing without Him. I am solely dependent on Him to anything including writing this book. Everything else is an illusion; the fact that you think you are doing anything on your own is an illusion. Either you are working for Him or the Dark One. Mammon or Yahuah?

I can't eat NATTO on my own. That is the power of the Holy One. I don't believe any of us can. I don't like being the bad guy to bring you this truth but this is my service to the Holy One. Otherwise, I'd be in big trouble myself if I kept this information to myself and joined the cowherd.

I want to be finished in this life with the acts of the Holy One. There is nothing I want more. I have had enough of this "WORLD" and the "THINGS" of it. But in order to live with Him I have to listen and obey and sometimes that "OBEYING" part can get a little uncomfortable. HalleluYAH!

Do you think Yahowashi was afraid of making people "uncomfortable" with his teachings?

Did He not tell it as it was even at the cost of his own life?

> If ye were of the world, the world would love his own: but because ye are not of the world, but I have chosen you out of the world, **Therefore the WORLD HATETH YOU.**
>
> John 15:19

All I know, is that I learn through trial and error and that I found if I listen and obey the Holy Spirit, I get well. And that's what I am encouraging you all to do. It's a lesson in obedience. That's all and everything else will be added unto you.

> But **seek** ye **first the Kingdom** of YAHUAH, and his righteousness; and all **the**se things shall be added unto you.
>
> Matthew 6:33

Are you living Righteously or are you living for self?

Are you living for others or are you living for self, family, and friends only?

It's all or nothing. There is no grey, in between. **Didn't Yahowashi say?**

So then because thou art lukewarm, and neither cold nor hot, **I WILL SPUE THEE OUT OF MY MOUTH.**

Revelation 3:16

These teachings are not just in the Bible, they are in every great literary work including the Bhagavad-Gita and the Master of Self-Realization and I am sure many others I don't yet know of. These teachings repeat themselves throughout history. Choose your guru/teacher and devote yourself unceasingly until you realize who you are. There is One Almighty God and there is Evil. Choose whom you will serve this day.

> And if it seem evil unto you to serve the LORD, choose you this day whom ye will serve; whether the gods which your fathers served that were on the other side of the flood, or the gods of the Amorites, in whose land ye dwell: but **as for me and my house, WE WILL SERVE the LORD.**
>
>
>
> **Joshua 24:15**
>
>

I found that when I tried to live by moderation, eating out only one time a week, very little meat, maybe some fish one a week, or a little coffee or chocolate one a week, I remained ill with recurrent skin lesion outbreaks but when I solely lived out of this world even solely eating for health, I became well and my lesions slowly began to cease.

Moderation is NOT the key, brothers and sisters, abstinence is and that goes for all pleasures of the flesh not just food. Then and only then will you be one with the Almighty God of the Universe and all things provided to you.

We cannot have "Pride of Life" and be one with the Almighty who gave us life. All things are provided for you when you surrender your life to Him and only Him. There are no in-betweens. It's only Him or nothing at all. HalleluYAH!

> **15 LOVE NOT the WORLD, neither the THINGS that are IN THE WORLD.** *If any man love the world*, **the LOVE of the Father is NOT in him.**
>
> **16** For ALL that is in the WORLD, the **LUST of the FLESH**, and the **LUST of the EYES,** and the **PRIDE of LIFE**, *is NOT of the Father,* **but is of the WORLD**.
>
> **17** And the WORLD PASSETH AWAY, and the LUST thereof: **but he that DOETH the WILL of God abideth forever.**
>
> **1 John 2:15-17**

Chapter 3

HOW TO MAKE JAPANESE NATTO

Making Japanese NATTO is rather simple. It takes a few tricks to make it just right but once you get the hang of it, it will become second nature.

- First Purchase Organic Soybeans and NATTO starter

  - I like Laura Organic Soybeans Organic Megumi Natto as both are U.S. sourced and very delicious

- Rinse Soybeans well

- Soak the beans 18-24 hours

  - Use 2 ½ parts distilled or filtered water to 1 part beans

- Rinse beans again

- Steam beans with pressure cooker on high 40-50 minutes

  - I cook 50 minutes as it makes for a nice soft bean once fermented

- Drain any excess water and place cooked beans into sterile glass dish

  - You can soak dish in hot soapy water or spray clean dish with rubbing alcohol

  - I cook the beans in the dish I used to soak, ferment, and store in by stacking two 6x6 inch square Pyrex in my pressure cooker. These dishes can only hold 1 cup dry beans each which expands to about 2 cups, or else it will spill over the top when cooking.

- Mix in about 1 heaping teaspoon full of NATTO starter into each dish you will be using and mix until all beans have come in contact with NATTO starter

- Next, this is very important, you will be placing two layers of clear plastic wrap over NATTO with tiny holes punched into the sheets of plastic to create an air pocket between the two sheets. A toothpick or fork may be used to make the holes. One sheet of plastic will be placed directly on-top of the beans after the holes have been made, the other sheet will be stretched tightly over the top edge of the dish to create the air pocket between the two sheets. Remember, both sheets should have holes punched through them at this point.

- Optional: I like to write on the top plastic wrap the words "LOVE NATTO HALLELUYAH," the date and time I placed into incubation, and any other variation I decided to try.

- Finally, place warm NATTO dishes into a large cooler bag wrapped in blankets or towels.

  o I use the large $7 cooler bags from Costco with a box placed on the bottom of it then cover NATTO with towels and blankets.

- Let the NATTO incubate 2-5 days. There should be a white halo around the beans seen through the glass and/or plastic wrap

- Store in the Refrigerator for up to 1-2 months. I like to start making a new batch when I am down to 1 dish of NATTO

Chapter 4

RECIPES IDEAS FOR NATTO

There are so many ways you can use NATTO.

- The traditional way is with sticky rice, mustard, soy sauce, and green Japanese onion. However, you could use radish sprouts, parsley, garlic, or any other herb and spices you prefer.

- You could make a smoothie with your favorite fruits and/or vegetables.

- Or perhaps a salad or soup such as miso and kelp soup.

- For myself, I prefer not to add heat to my NATTO as it seems to lessen its unique characteristics that I feel are most beneficial to our health.

I will leave the creating up to you. I find that it's not so much how you eat it, but that you eat it.

Other food supplements I find helpful are:

- CELTIC SEA SALT as it has three different types of Magnesium among 82 other essential minerals our body needs, and is the only salt that alkalizes the body.
- MAIN COAST SEA VEGETABLES from Iceland and Sea Kelp to get our much needed iodine.
- And if anyone is in pain, I find that Kannaway has the BEST CBD OIL ON EARTH; one of the products I like best is the REVIVE PRO with added Chinese Bibong herbs which seems to enhance the effectiveness. Please contact me if you are interested in purchasing.

I hope you all have found this information beneficial and will empower you to be in good health. May YAHUAH bless you all.

12 *Beloved,* **think it NOT strange** *concerning* **the fiery trial** *which* **is to try you**, *as though some strange thing happened unto you.*

¹³ **BUT REJOICE!** *Inasmuch* **as ye are partakers of HaMashiach's sufferings;** *THAT, when His GLORY shall be revealed,* **ye may BE GLAD also with EXCEEDING JOY!**

1 Peter 4:12-13

BECAUSE:

The sacrifices of YAHUAH are a broken spirit: a broken and a contrite heart, *O YAHUAH, thou wilt not despise.*

Psalm 51:17

¹⁸ **The LORD hath chastened me sore**: <u>*BUT*</u> **He hath NOT given me over unto Death**. *[HALLELUYAH!]*

THEREFORE:

¹⁷ **I SHALL not die, but LIVE, and DECLARE the WORKS of the LORD.**

Psalm 118:18, 17

¹⁸ **I counsel thee to buy of me GOLD TRIED IN THE FIRE**, *that thou* **mayest be rich;** *and* **WHITE**

29

RAIMENT, *that thou* **mayest be clothed,** *and that* **the shame of thy nakedness do not appear;** *and* **ANOINT THINE EYES with eyesalve,** *that thou* **mayest see.**

¹⁹ **As many as I LOVE, I REBUKE and CHASTEN: BE ZEALOUS** *therefore,* **and REPENT.**

²⁰ **BEHOLD, I STAND AT THE DOOR, AND KNOCK:** IF ANY MAN HEAR MY VOICE, AND OPEN THE DOOR, **I will come in to him, and will sup with him, and he with me.**

Revelation 3:18-20

And **they overcame him [EVIL/SIN/SATAN]:**

1) *by the BLOOD of the Lamb,* AND

2) *by the WORD of their TESTIMONY;*

3) **AND they LOVED <u>NOT</u> their LIVES UNTO the DEATH.**

Revelation 12:11

ABOUT THE AUTHOR

Victoria Bell is a Registered Nurse, author, lecturer passionate about empowering others find TRUE FREEDOM, PEACE, and RESTORATION from any DIS-EASE through Spiritual Healing and Practical Application.

We Believe in Miracles
Because We Believe in YAHUAH!
HalleluYAH!!

Thank you for Joining Us!

If you have been blessed by this book, please bless us with a positive review and by sharing your Testimony on Amazon.com
Thank You!

Additional Copies of this Book are Available on **Amazon.com**

NOTES

_____

_____

_____

_____

_____

_____

_____

_____

Hallelujah! YAHUAH LOVES Me!

_____

_____

_____

_____

_____

_____

_____

_____

_____

_____

Hallelujah! YAHUAH LOVES Me!

_____

_____

_____

_____

_____

_____

_____

_____

_____

_____

Hallelujah! YAHUAH LOVES Me!

_____

_____

_____

_____

_____

_____

_____

_____

_____

_____

Hallelujah! YAHUAH LOVES Me!

Printed in Great Britain
by Amazon

22843509R00020